POWER YOUR BODY

While enjoying your present lifestyle

Curion

DEDICATION

Dedicated to the memory of my loving Dad
and to my Mom who continues to inspire me
with her values

ACKNOWLEDGEMENTS

Printed by CreateSpace,
An Amazon.com Company

CONTENTS

Dedication iii

Acknowledgements i

Contents ii

Preface 1

1. Introduction 6

What is meant by 'Powering Your Body'? 7

Why do we interfere with the body functions?................8

What are we going to do?...............................9

Nature is the best teacher..............................9

Have you thought about these?..........................10

What do we need to do?.................................10

How is this book written? 11

What this book is about and what it is not.....................11

2. The Structure of Life 13

What we eat is what we gets 13

The balance in the body 15

The parts of the body 15

The Gases 17

The Heat 18

The Liquids...20

The Interaction of Heat, Liquids and Gases...............22

What will be the effect of their imbalance? 23

3. Taste and how to use it to help us.................................28

Characteristics of Sweet Taste. 29

Characteristics of Sour Taste 31

Characteristics of Salty Taste 33

Characteristics of Pungent Taste................................34

Characteristics of Bitter Taste 35

Characteristics of Astringent Taste................................36

Overview of the use of taste 38

4. Origin and Properties of materials 41

Thriving in Water 42

Living in Wetland 45

Dry-land 46

Desert.................................47

Mountain and Forests.................................48

Icy Terrains.................................49

5. Signs and Solutions 52

Pain 52

Taste 53

Tiredness.................................53

Irritability 54

Confusion 54

Laziness.................................55

Sleepiness.................................56

Sleeplessness.................................56

Memory 57

Climate tolerance 58

Emotion 59

6. The Invisible Forces 62

Positive and Negative Forces. 62

Opposite and complementary. 63

Interdependent for equilibrium. 64

The duality of human body 64

Common deficiency and excess of the forces 65

7. Notice to your Body 68

Sight 68

Touch 69

Sound 69

Smell 69

Taste 70

8. Golden Rules for Good Health 72

9. Mental Health 76

10. Summary 80

ABOUT THE AUTHOR 82

PREFACE

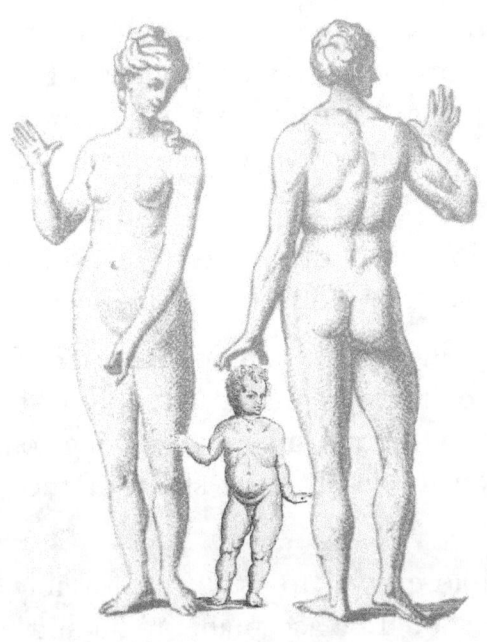

We are going to explore the long forgotten truths about the human body. The human body is a versatile instrument with an intricate system of mechanisms.

It is deceptively simple looking but anyone studying its physiology or morphology would feel perplexed at the degree of complexity it gets into.

The body and mind work synchronously and affect each other. The mind has a strong influence on the body and many physiological changes were made possible by changing the perceptions of the mind according physicians as well as psychologists.

We also know that drugs given to the body have an effect on the mind as well

There is an endless debate about which system of medicine and healing is better, which drugs are good and which ones have side effects and which ones are toxic.

New inventions in the field of health and wellness reveal changing and often contradicting views of physicians and scientists. There are also controversies about the methods of healing and nutrition and the resultant physical and mental well being.

There are different health systems as wide as the world from East to West or North to South.

We are not going via the traditional scientific or medical route. We won't go to the magic and mystic territories either. We won't accept anything defying logic. Our goal here would be to simplify the study of the body and its mechanisms.

We would explore a way to use it comfortably and usefully. This method should be acceptable to all and practicable to all.

Pediatric therapy is different from Geriatric treatment. This is because the body of a child and that of an elderly person differ in many respects.

We would try to find out what is common in all the human bodies and how it functions irrespective of age, gender, ethnicity and other factors.

There may be nothing in this book that a common person cannot understand.

This book is based on my personal study and research in to various subjects like medicinal systems, herbs, minerals, therapies, nutrition, properties of materials, physics, chemistry, biology, yoga, meditation, spiritual subjects, culture and religion, and alternative approaches to wellness.

My three decades of experience with my family members, my friends, relatives, and my own body with respect to wellness, nutrition and therapy were very valuable in making such an analysis possible. The observations shared here are not just theoretical but based on my real experience as well.

There have been enormous changes in science and technology, languages, culture, politics, social makeup and everything one can think of during the centuries. Yet the core principles of 'life' and the biological system of the human body remain the same.

There are changes of evolution and adaptation of the body to changing ambiances but the basic philosophy is a constant.

We can change the containers, method of cooking and the presentation but we can only eat food and nothing else.

We can wear any kind of dress, live in any kind of house, use any instrument and travel by any kind of vehicle but we cannot get rid of the body.

The concept of life is embedded in this body. It has built in rules and regulations irrespective if you prefer to call them as DNA or anything else. If we try to meddle with its natural working order we would end up unsuccessful.

We can accomplish nothing by taking a contradictory approach to our bodies. If we can identify a way to align our preferences with the body's own order, then we can influence the body's behavior.

This book is intended to kindle your thinking and make you aware of your surroundings and how the world affects your life and wellness. That way you can find a method that suits you and makes you feel comfortable.

You are unique and your body is unique. You need a unique approach to maintain it and live a healthy and happy life.

1. INTRODUCTION

You don't have to be a physician to observe your own body. But it requires some practice to understand and interpret the body's subtle and overt messages.

We would try to delve into this field. We can cure ourselves from illness using these methods.

They would also help the physician in properly diagnosing the illness by providing the relevant information about the symptoms.

> *I don't recommend here any medicines - Allopathy, Homeopathy, Naturopathy, Ayurveda, Chinese Medicine, or any other system.*
>
> *I don't advise you to do any strenuous exercise, gym, tread mill or workout.*
>
> *I don't also suggest any nutritional supplements, herbs, or anything bizarre.*

The efficacy of the above methods differs from system to system and from person to person. I am not elaborating anything about this mysterious territory.

The skills of the physician are, in my humble opinion, more important than the system of medicine or the drugs prescribed. This is more so in systems where the drugs and the methods of application have not been standardized. (like in Ayurveda, Unani, Chinese medicine and some holistic systems).

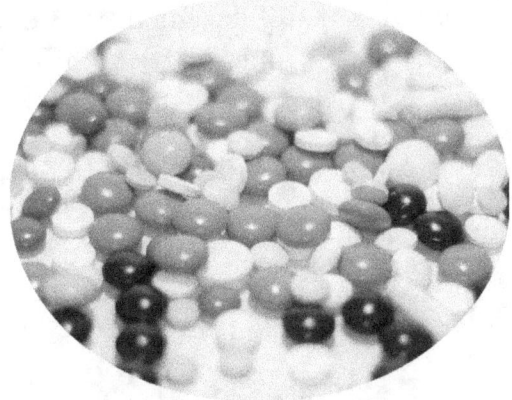

No particular system of medicine and nutrition can be considered the safest, most effective and therefore the best. Many physicians tend to treat their patients symptomatically to be on the safe side.

What I suggest here is a system of consciously watching your body and mind and following simple dos and don'ts.

You don't need to change your lifestyle unless it is erratic or abnormal.

The best part is you cannot damage yourself by using these methods.

WHAT IS MEANT BY 'POWERING YOUR BODY'?

Does your body have no power? It sure has its natural powers. The moment we are born the body starts to function by itself. It can take care of itself. But it needs the assistance of its parts to function properly.

When it needs food, it intimates the hands to feed, the mouth to crush and swallow and also instructs the digestive system to assimilate.

All the body functions are designed to be carried out automatically. But these functions are affected by our actions.

Powering the body is actually empowering the body to regain its 'control over itself'. We do this by reducing our interference with its system.

WHY DO WE INTERFERE WITH THE BODY FUNCTIONS?

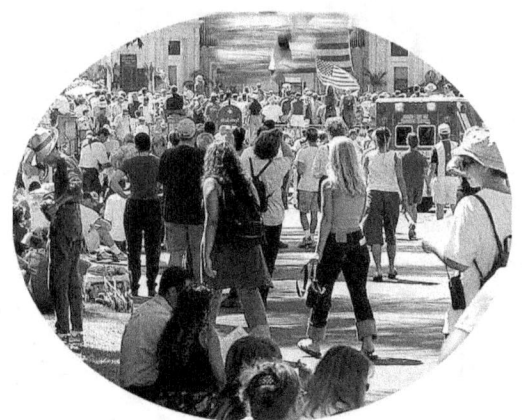

We impose on the body certain conditions and restrictions that we think we are comfortable with or that we consider better for us. This can be due to our lifestyle, habits, work conditions, economic factors and external atmosphere. Our perception of good health, social factors, stresses, strain and abnormal demands on the body also matter.

These stresses put a burden on the body to over work and the body has to adjust itself to these abuses.

The constraints that prevent the normal functioning of the body need to be corrected.

The body has to regain its freedom.

WHAT ARE WE GOING TO DO?

We are going to use an empirical approach. We would simply try to manage our food, activity and rest.

We would explore how to tune our body and mind. We are going to do that in such a way that our physical and mental comforts are the least modified.

It would be easy to follow.

It would be suitable for all ages.

NATURE IS THE BEST TEACHER

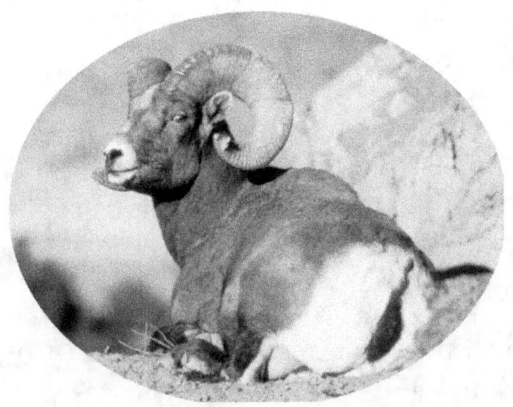

Watch the animals. They don't exercise. They are almost always fit. They rarely fall ill. Have you wondered why? They don't consciously take care of their bodies. Rather they go with the natural order.

They are not as intelligent as humans. That is their blessing. They don't assume that their knowledge is superior to the body's own knowledge of itself. They are not invasive like us in treating the body.

HAVE YOU THOUGHT ABOUT THESE?

Wild animals don't go to a hospital to deliver babies. They don't have a physician to look after them.

You accidentally cut your finger with a knife but you don't apply any medicine. A man gets a cut while having a shave. These wounds heal themselves.

You swallow some toxic substance. The body protects you by inducing vomiting and throwing the unwanted stuff.

You don't need to instruct the body to protect itself from such difficulties.

You just need to leave it by itself or support it if possible as described later in this book.

WHAT DO WE NEED TO DO?

We would try to stop anything that disrupts the normal functioning of the body. We would try to aid the body in its smooth functioning.

To accomplish this, a clear understanding of hygiene, food, body functions and the mental process is all that is required.

We would be using the natural diagnostic tools present in our own bodies.

We would be listening to their warnings and messages. It is not as tough as it sounds.

We just need to re-learn what we forgot in the course of our busy lives.

Our aim is to reclaim the full potential of the body.

A study is also made of some treatments to relieve ailments to know how to keep ourselves fit with optimum health.

HOW IS THIS BOOK WRITTEN?

We would be studying about the body and the mind.

We will explore what is the system, how is it organized and how does it function.

We will study about what can go wrong with the system, why and when.

We would analyze how to reset it back to its original state.

WHAT THIS BOOK IS ABOUT AND WHAT IT IS NOT

This book is intended to provide information about the human body to stimulate your thinking and create awareness about possible abuse of your body.

Easy non invasive methods without any adverse side effects have been presented.

I don't prescribe or advise you to follow anything contained in this book. If it makes sense, try it. You may follow them at your own free will.

Please note that this book is not a treatise on medicine or therapy.

The advice of a qualified physician should be sought for any kind of illness.

It is my disclaimer that I cannot be held responsible for any of your actions relating to this .information whatsoever.

2. THE STRUCTURE OF LIFE

Any living being eats something, uses some of it, and discards the rest. What we eat is known as food, it is the input. It can be of plant, animal or mineral origin.

The food is converted into body tissues like flesh, blood, or bones. Some components of the food are not converted but they aid in the conversion of other particles. Some other parts are not useful to us and they are simply excreted.

The ingredients remaining after assimilation are discarded as waste. The worn out parts of the body tissues are also discarded as waste. This renewal and rebuilding is a continuous process.

WHAT WE EAT IS WHAT WE GETS

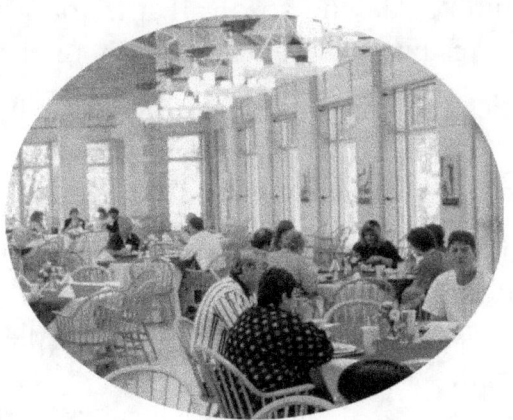

The items we eat have their own physical and chemical properties. For example, they are red, yellow, hard, soft, sweet, sour, nice smelling, pungent, light, heavy, soluble in water, dry, wet, oily, carbohydrates, proteins, fibers, antioxidants, moisturizers and so on.

It is only natural that 'we absorb these properties' when we eat the ingredients which contain them.

Put some sugar into water and it becomes sweet. As long as a little sugar is present in the water it would be sweet.

What we eat makes up our body. Sounds logical? Right, we shall see how we are using use this concept every day in our lives.

We take a leaf or other part of a plant and find out what are the components it contains, like proteins, carbohydrates or chlorophyll.

We may also take a bit of a mineral and research what happens if we eat it. We find out what each of these components do in our body.

If we can figure out what effect it has on our body, we call it a nutritional ingredient. We name these components as vitamins, amino acids and so on. If it is found to be more aggressive, we call it a drug and use it as a medicine.

The properties of these materials affect our body, for the good or for the bad. Likewise, animal matter and mineral particles also have some action on the body.

Not only what we eat but also what we apply on the skin, or inhale through our noses, or connect with our body in any manner has some physiological action. Allergies can be cited as examples.

The study of interaction of materials with our body is known as pharmacology. Many of us may know this fact but are not always conscious of this.

THE BALANCE IN THE BODY

When you ride a bicycle, you match your tilt to the right and left, control the speed and adjust your posture so that you are stable and do not fall. We match the gravity, wind, forward thrust and other forces. We call this as balancing. To keep going you need to balance.

Similarly in order to keep the body functioning, we need to keep it in balance.

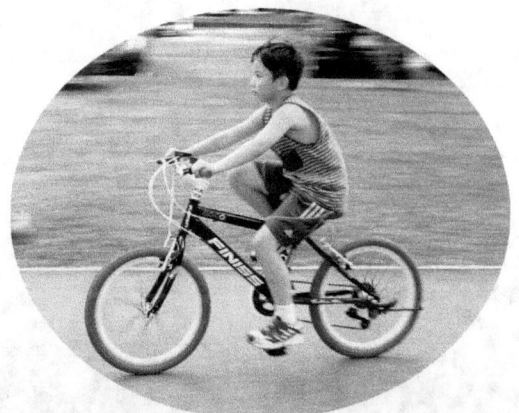

What do we balance? We should first find out what are the forces in the body that are in balance. This is an abstract understanding, so please think carefully.

Is it the heart rate or pulse? Is it the number of respirations per minute? Is it the blood pressure? Is it how many times you urinate or defecate? Is it the height to weight ratio? Is it the body mass index? Or should you use the more exotic term known as biorhythm? These are symptoms caused by the forces.

THE PARTS OF THE BODY

Do we know the parts of the body? Are they the eyes, ears, arms, intestines and all that? Here we would classify the parts differently. Instead of identifying a part based on its form or appearance, we classify them into groups based on their properties and functions.

We can classify them as the respiratory system, the digestive system, the circulatory system, the nervous system, the excretory system or the reproductive system.

It is more meaningful. This type of classification is more integrating. It does not divide the body into disjointed parts.

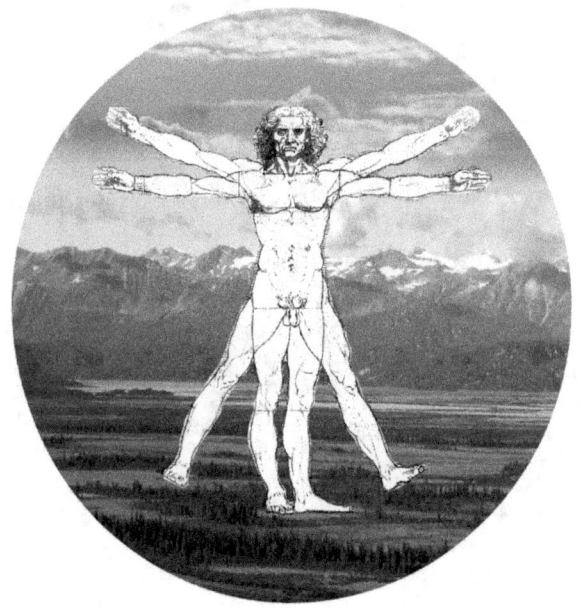

We can also divide them into broad elemental groups. Some parts of the body are solid like the bone and hair. Some others are liquid like blood, saliva and urine. There are gases in the body. Some are hot.

There are five universal elements known as Earth, Water, Fire, Gases and Space. Out of these five elements, we can understand that Earth and Space are both seemingly stationary, while the remaining three namely Gases, Fire and Water are mobile.

For our study, we are interested in classifying the body components into three types - Gases, Heat, and Liquids.

We select these because they are active, mobile and changing.

Solids and Space change in a very subtle manner and therefore it would be very difficult for us to observe their activities.

We use this system of dividing the body because it would be easy to observe them 'in action'. We would also be able to make intentional changes to them.

The Indian system of medicine known as Ayurveda takes in to account these three elements and terms them as Vata, Pitta and Kapha respectively.

THE GASES

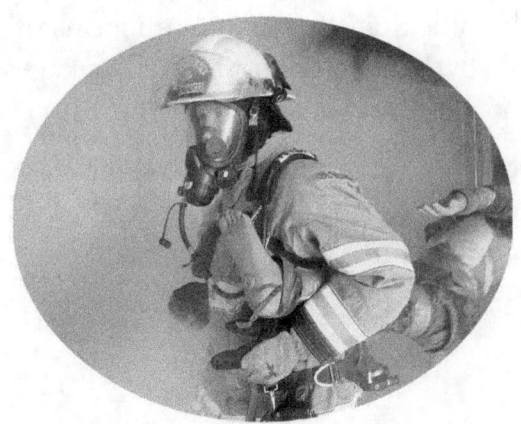

They can be beneficial. Oxygen with a little moisture is beneficial to the body. Some vapors are considered good if they aid in the alleviation of diseases or removal of waste from the body.

They are also good if they reduce the pain and suffering. Oxygen is needed throughout our body. The body tries to inhale and absorb good gases. Not only the lungs but the whole body including our skin absorbs gases as well.

The gases can be bad. High amounts of water vapor and Carbon Dioxide are bad for the body.

Many toxic and poisonous gases are dangerous if inhaled or contacted. Carbon dioxide is exhaled through the lungs along with water vapor and waste gases.

Flatus also contains degraded particles and biological matter which have been converted into gas. Undigested food and some decayed cells are converted to gas and expelled from the body.

Gases are more mobile than liquids and can quickly move from one part to another part. They can penetrate the body cells very easily through the minute pores.

If unwanted gas is not removed from the body it creates discomfort by blocking the normal functions of that part. It can be especially felt in functions such as digestion, blood circulation, mobility and action of the limbs.

If a gas is not good for the body it usually has an offensive or pungent odour and the gases beneficial to the body have a pleasant aroma and people are comfortable with their smell.

THE HEAT

Heat is present in our body when we are alive and cools off when we are dead. There is continuous burning of fuel in the body and this is the source of heat. When there is more activity in the body, there would be a lot of combustion.

During times of infection the body fights germs and there is hyper activity going on. The heat would be great which we call as fever.

The active part of a body would be hot and the inactive part would be cold. The hot part would also indicate the heat by a red color. The cooler parts would be bluish.

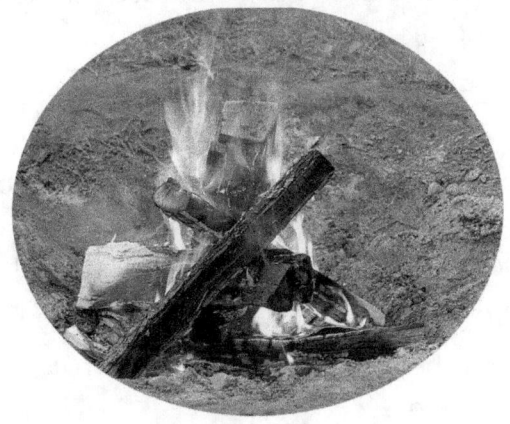

There is a vital heat of the body which is responsible for the digestion of food. It is also responsible for the distribution of the fuel or energy to different parts of the body.

You can easily observe the heat in your body when you fall sick.

If you are happy and excited the heat raises as does the blood pressure. The harder you work the more heat is generated.

To cool the body to its normal temperature you perspire. The sweating is the function of the heat-exchanger of the body that is the skin.

If there is heat there is activity, movement, transformation and well being. Coolness indicates the opposite, which is inaction, numbness, decay, illness and ultimately death.

The extremes of heat and cool are not good for the body.

Heat is generated by fire which in turn needs fuel to burn. Without fuel fire will extinguish. Lack of fuel at the required location can be a reason for reduced activity at any part of the body.

This phenomenon mostly goes unnoticed while we think of discomforts and disabilities.

THE LIQUIDS

Water is the major liquid component of the body. Many substances dissolve in water. We use water to clean articles and wash clothes. We also use water to dissolve materials for easier application.

Likewise water helps to dissolve good particles and bad particles in the body.

Watery liquids also perform similar tasks. Liquids help to absorb the energy giving particles and other good materials like medicines and nutrients and assist in transporting them to needed parts of the body.

Without the aid of liquids all the parts of the body will not receive the nutrients and energy.

They cannot be treated of infections without the help of liquids to deliver the drugs to the required cell.

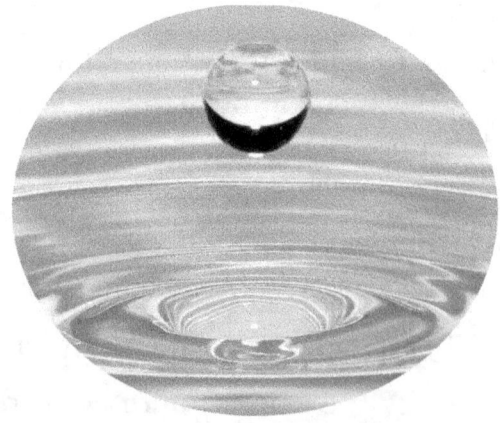

Certain liquids cannot be converted in to gas for transport to different parts for effective use by the body. These have to be necessarily transported in the liquid phase.

Some liquids will have dissolved and suspended solids in them.

Most of the nutrients required by the body are kept and used in the liquid form.

Liquids also help perform the very important function of removal of wastes and toxics from the body.

Urine and sweat remove the wastes dissolved in liquids. Vomiting removes any toxic substances accidentally swallowed into the stomach.

Blood, lymph, inter-cellular fluids, semen, and hormones are all liquids. They have to travel great distances within the body cavities at a quick pace and on demand.

We can say that liquids are the most important of the three components we have taken up for study. Liquid state is the best state for these fluids to perform their intended functions.

Human beings can survive without food for some time but not without water.

The Interaction of Heat, Liquids and Gases

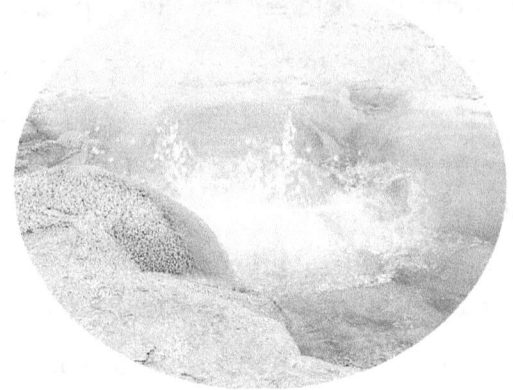

Gases, heat and liquids present in the body cannot thrive in isolation. They have to contact each other at various places in the body. In fact they depend on each other for their normal functioning. It is essential that they are compatible with each other in every respect.

Natural hot water springs generate hot water and steam which make them to move from one place to another.

In our body too some of the liquids may get converted into gases in the course of the body processes. This is how gas troubles develop. Heat and inflammation may result during such processes.

The Gases, Heat and Liquids in the body should be at balance. Otherwise they create weakness and allow diseases and disabilities to develop.

WHAT WILL BE THE EFFECT OF THEIR IMBALANCE?

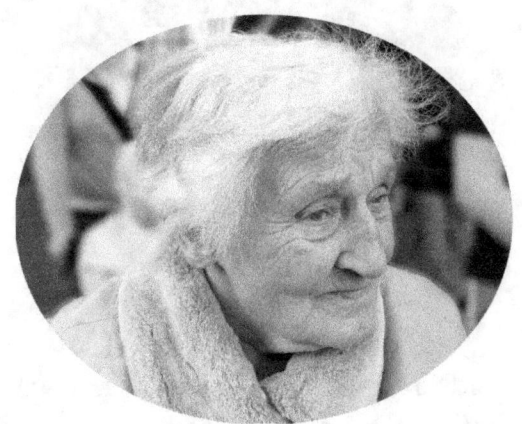

Inadequacy of liquids causes dryness. The body has less than the optimum quantity of water and other liquids.

The body feels hot, dry, shrunk, dull, and the skin lacks luster. The body suffers from watery eyes, constipation, less or more urination, bladder irritation, thirst, sleeplessness, tiredness and general inertia.

Mental symptoms of insufficient liquids would be haste, irritability, lack of concentration, confusion, and inability to think clearly.

There may be an inclination to resort to alcohol and drugs.

What causes such a condition? Consuming more dry and fried foods or generally dehydrated food rather than boiled or steamed food is a predominant reason.

Starving and Mal-nutrition are the other causes. Exposure to extreme cold and hot climates, lack of physical activity or laziness also create such a condition.

When these symptoms are seen one should consume more water, liquids, and fruits.

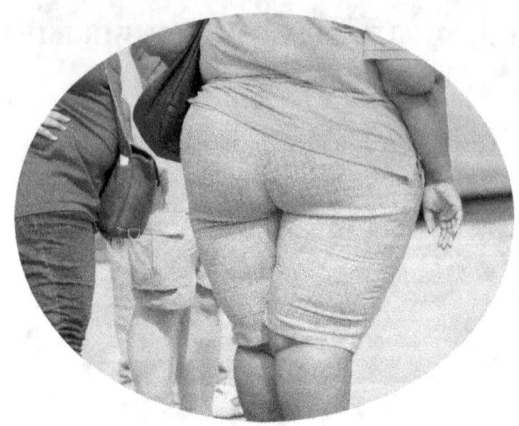

Excess of liquids results in obesity, weight gain, frequent sweating, urination, higher blood pressure, desire to sleep and lethargy. Reducing liquid intake and increasing heat as described below may be beneficial.

Less than optimum heat can result in indigestion, visual impairment, cold, cough and respiratory infections, lack of interest in sex, reduced appetite or even aversion to food, acidity and regurgitation, sleepiness and general inertia.

Eating stale, cold food, eating at irregular intervals, sleep deprivation, lack of physical activity, consuming more starchy and fatty foods are some of the causes.

For some persons mental illusions and hallucinations can be felt.

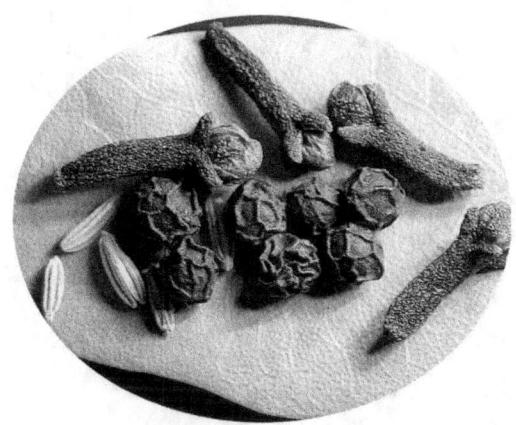

To set it right one should take carminatives and hot spices like pepper or ginger. Eat only fresh hot food. Avoid cool drinks, ice-cream, and fruits.

Mild physical exercises would enable the body processes to resume.

Breathing exercises would also be beneficial by activating the stomach muscles.

Alcohol in small amounts might help in producing some heat. Cold drinks, green vegetables and salads should be avoided.

Excess heat shows the same symptoms as inadequate liquids along with increased thirst and hunger.

It can be compensated by consuming liquids, fruits and vegetables and taking moderate rest.

When gases are below or above the balanced levels, the symptoms would be: pain in extremities, inability to properly use arms and legs, flatus, quick temper, impatience, indigestion, lack of appetite or feeling of vomiting, feeling cold and even shivering, fear of death or inability, headache, dizziness, erratic blood pressure, nervousness, sleeplessness and hair loss.

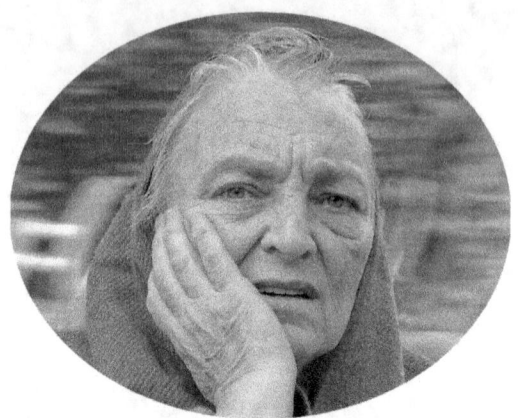

Causes include more fatty and spicy diet, excessive eating, excessive alcohol and lack of physical activity.

Remedial measures to take are regular exercise or at least a walk every day. Correct your food according to your digestive capacity.

It would better to keep warm, avoid exposure to extreme cold, take sunbath, massage the body with warm oils and eat only hot freshly prepared foods.

We so far studied how the five elements of the universe function in our own bodies.

Next we shall explore how to use our senses to aid in the diagnosis and to keep fit.

3. TASTE AND HOW TO USE IT TO HELP US

Tastes are considered very valuable to diagnose and treat illness in Ayurveda and other eastern systems of medicine (India, China and Japan).

Homeopathy also studies the change in taste perceptions and treats the patient accordingly.

Anyone can use taste as a diagnostic tool. It can also be used to select the range of food items that can be advantageously consumed.

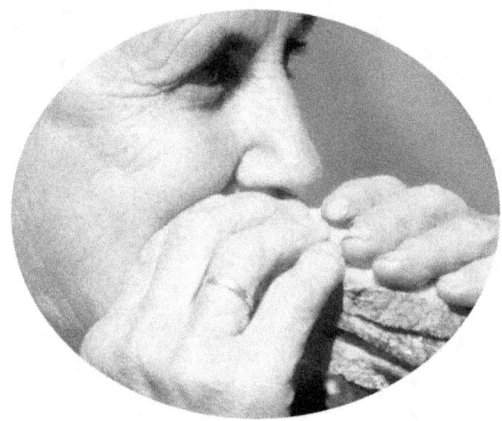

Taste sends information to the body about the kind of food we are eating and the body responds by secreting the appropriate enzymes to digest that particular food.

It would also prepare to take care of any adverse actions the food might have on the body.

Taste is an indication and warning mechanism to our digestive and metabolic system.

You can see people salivating on seeing and tasting some food. There are also other glands which produce different liquids as a response to the taste which we do not normally observe.

There is also a message to our mind embedded in the taste signal.

Materials which are sweet, sour, salty, bitter, pungent, and astringent have different properties. We may feel that the taste is fatty, dry, nauseating or itching also.

They clearly indicate the action of these substances on our body.

Sweet substances are considered good while bitter ones are usually thought of as poisons. They may be accompanied by offensive odors.

By choosing the foodstuff that tastes good and by avoiding those that are of bad taste and disagree with our body (for example, creating indisposition or allergies), we can lead a healthy life.

CHARACTERISTICS OF SWEET TASTE.

This is the most sought after taste among all humans and also the most beneficial one to the body.

Sweet associates itself with building body tissues, tones nerves and brain and provides stamina.

Sweet taste is the manifestation of Water and Earth of the five universal elements.

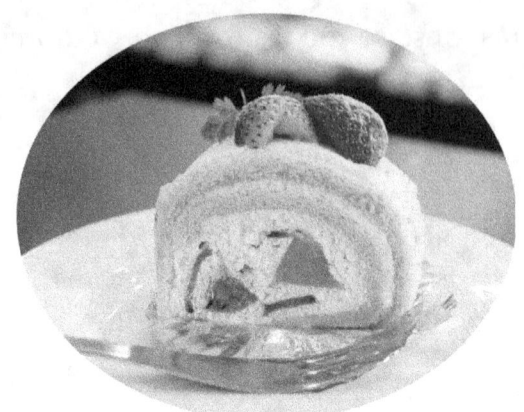

Even a newborn baby is involuntarily drawn towards things which are sweet.

Consuming and sharing sweets promotes a sense of well being and acts as a psychological boost. We tend to celebrate occasions with sweet.

Many animals too have a preference to things which are sweet.

Sweet is indeed good for the body. The body's energy is stored as a sweet substance known as glucose. Carbohydrates in the form of starch are converted into sugars in the body before it is used.

Any sweet can be a handy and instant energy to the human body especially in times of distress. It is a store of energy.

Sweet taste denotes the highest energy density.

Sweet can preserve many nutrients, vitamins, minerals and medicinal substances for long.

Some valuable medical substances are available in nature as their sugar compounds.

Sweet provides mass to the tissues, moisturises it and cools the body. It produces, blood, plasma, bone marrow, semen, saliva, albumin and mucous membranes.

It is a mark of vitality and robust health.

Grains, fat, proteins, beans, lentils, fruits, carrots, beets, potatoes, sugars and milk are some food items which are sweet.

Sometimes the sweet taste is delicate and would be revealed only after some chewing in the mouth.

Sweet food and beverages are beneficial to those who are weak, convalescing, lean and emaciated. It would help persons who lack normal physical and mental growth or have physical deformities.

It cures acidity and metabolic disorders, constipation, gastric troubles, many types of headaches and dizziness, stress related symptoms, ulcer, cancer, tumour, and dehydrated body and skin.

Eating sweet food should be limited by those who have skin infections, respiratory disorders, obesity, sleepiness, drowsiness, excessive urination, unexplained infections, diseases of the reproductive organs and dental problems.

Sweet need not be avoided except in extreme cases.

CHARACTERISTICS OF SOUR TASTE

This taste is the second in the order of energy density and denotes the presence of acids. The acids may be inorganic or organic.

Some of these are essential for our digestion and protection from harmful organisms.

Sour taste serves as an appetizer. It quenches thirst.

Substances having a sour taste like lime, mango and tamarind can be used as preservatives to prolong shelf life of food items.

Sour milk like yogurt, cheese, fermented items like wine, vinegar, pickles and soy sauce are commonly used in every household.

Sour taste is the manifestation of Earth and Fire of the five elements.

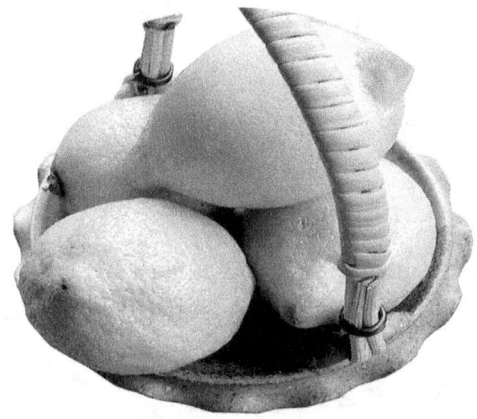

Sour substances help blood circulation, strengthen the heart and sharpen the senses.

They can be advantageous to relieve nauseating sensation.

Natural sour acids extract minerals and medicinal active principles from vegetable and animal matter and make them available to the body.

It also helps to dissolve toxins and waste products in water to be excreted as urine.

The acidic nature kills the bacteria and other germs present in the digestive tract especially the stomach and urinary bladder.

Fruits and vegetables having sour taste are generally rich in Vitamin C and are important for resistance to diseases.

In moderate quantities they promote digestion but if consumed in excess sour articles cause acidity and ulcers.

This taste is associated with feminine nature as described later here.

CHARACTERISTICS OF SALTY TASTE

Natural salts extracted from the sea and rocks as also some substances obtained from plant origin have this kind of taste known as salty.

There may be slight differences between the tastes of substances. For instance, Sodium salts taste differently from Potassium or Magnesium salts.

Salty taste connotes lesser energy density than sourness.

It manifests the Fire and Water of the elements.

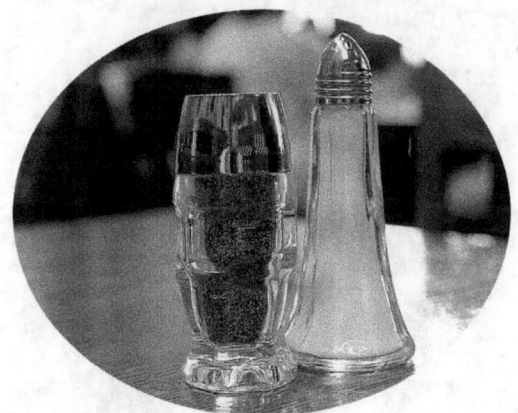

They are neutral or alkaline in nature.

The substances having salty to bland taste are considered masculine in nature by many alternative medical systems.

It has water retaining qualities, maintains mineral and electrolyte balance in the body, soothes nervous systems and promotes growth.

CHARACTERISTICS OF PUNGENT TASTE

This taste is characterised by irritation and heat as is felt when tasting substances like pepper, chilies and ginger.

The foods having such a taste are medium in their energy densities.

These substances are carminatives and help in the secretion of digestive juices in the body.

They also generate heat in the body. They alleviate pain, disability, and some other kinds of illness.

External application provides heat to the limbs which have gone numb due to exposure to cold temperatures.

They also provide symptomatic relief from inflammation of the limbs due to injuries.

It promotes perspiration and eliminates excess gas from the body.

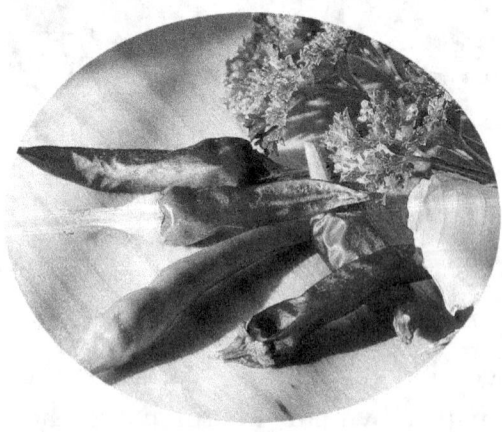

Pungent taste manifests from the Fire and Air of the five elements.

Pungent tasting materials aid in removing blocks to blood circulation and kindle the nervous system to help recovering from diseases such as blood clot and paralysis.

They generally increase the blood pressure and circulation.

CHARACTERISTICS OF BITTER TASTE

They shrink the cells of the body and try to dry them.

They increase the vital heat of the body.

They enhance eye sight and provide a glow to the skin by making it opaque.

They are germicidal in nature and also repel most of the organisms in the body.

They help to reduce the moisture in the body and thus reduce weight.

They also reduce the blood sugar levels in human beings.

When taken raw or in sufficient quantities, bitters act as a de-worming agents to get rid of intestinal parasites.

External application of bitters like neem has been found to cure skin eruptions and chicken pox.

They act as mosquito and other insect repellents.

Bitter taste forms out of the manifestation of Air and Space.

Many poisonous and toxic substances are bitter in taste.

Bitter taste is detected by the tongue very easily even in minute quantities. This capability of the tongue may be a mechanism built in to our body for warning and protection.

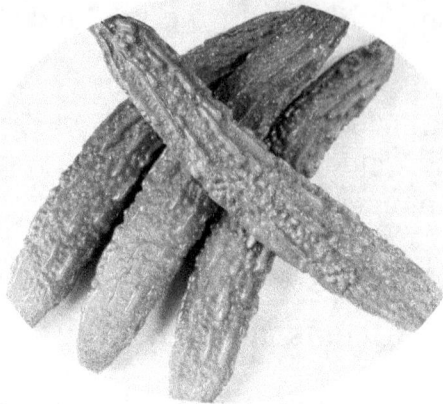

However, not all bitters are bad. Some bitters like Quinine and Neem have been used as potent medicines for many centuries.

Ancient medical practitioners used even poisonous bitters in low doses to cure chronic diseases.

Some old time texts describe a few bitters as Elixirs of Life and as cure-all medicines.

CHARACTERISTICS OF ASTRINGENT TASTE

This taste is akin to bitter but without the unpleasantness. They leave a dry and rough feeling on the tongue.

This taste also denotes that the substance would contract the cells and tissues and slightly dehydrate.

They relieve cough and cold since they act readily on the mucous substances.

They are general antiseptics. The substances of this taste are applied topically on wounds as an antiseptic and also to heal them.

They are considered as a good remedy for diarrhea.

They are used to cure sore throat and hemorrhages.

They condition the oily skin.

Some eye lotions contain astringents which are non-irritating and cool. Nasal and Ear drops too contain astringents.

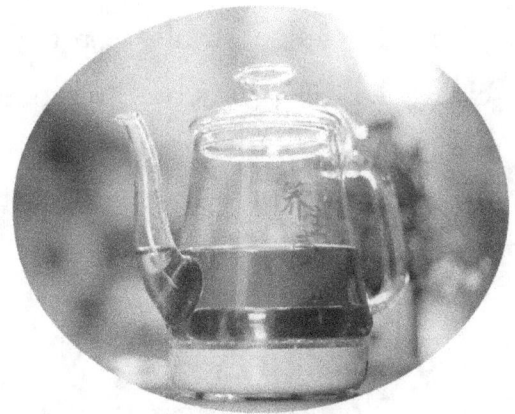

Some substances having an astringent taste are coffee, tea, raw pears, pomegranate, and rye.

This taste removes the slimy feeling in the mouth and makes it feel dry and rough. Due to this property they are incorporated in dental preparations from historical times.

It manifests from Air and Earth of the five elements.

In eastern medical systems they are used to tighten sagging muscles in elderly persons. Ground paste of astringent materials was applied to the skin to clear wrinkles.

They are also associated with long life.

OVERVIEW OF THE USE OF TASTE

Taste: **SWEET**

Found in: Milk, grains, legumes, fruits, carrot.

Good for: Weight gain, energy, nerves, reproduction, hair, voice.

Bad for: Respiratory infections, obesity, urinary and skin diseases.

Taste: **SOUR**

Found in: Lemon, Yogurt, Vinegar, Soy sauce, Mango, Tamarind.

Good for: Vitamin C source, digestion, thirst, vision.

Bad for: Acidity, male impotence, ulcers, tumors.

Taste: **SALTY**

Found in: Sea salt, leafy vegetables, stems of plants, mineral salts.

Good for: Antacids, nutrients dissolution, fluid thickness, body bulk, lymph.

Bad for: Female impotence, anemia, menstrual problems, gray hair.

Taste: **PUNGENT**

Found in: Chillies, pepper, garlic, onion, ginger, cloves, mustard.

Good for: Relieves indigestion, cramps, detoxification, cold, cough, muscular pain.

Bad for: Ulcer, acidity, loose stools, dehydration, convalescing, weakness.

Taste: **BITTER**

Found in: Fenugreek, bitter gourd, turmeric, olive, grapefruit.

Good for: Diabetes, detoxifying, anti-biotic, obesity reduction, skin diseases.

Bad for: Metabolic disorders, hepatitis, physical disabilities, weakness.

Taste: **ASTRINGENT**

Found in: Coffee, tea, pomegranate, alum, alcohol.

Good for: Cold, cough, bleeding, diarrhea, ulcers, tighten muscles.

Bad for: Dry skin, weakness, gastric problems.

4. ORIGIN AND PROPERTIES OF MATERIALS

Let us study the properties of animals, plants and minerals originating from various places on the earth.

We shall look at what are the differentiating factors in each of their physical systems.

This study would be helpful because our food always consists of materials derived from animals, plants and minerals.

A careful analysis of their characteristics would help us to decide which food is beneficial to our present state of health and which would be detrimental to our body.

Generally speaking we have to take a 'complementary and compensatory' approach in choosing our foodstuff.

A person living in a dry area will naturally lack nutrients of things found in water. Similarly one living in a wet place would need nutrients found in the desert.

A fat person requires the substances available from lean objects and a lean person needs the nutrients of a fat object.

Here is an example I am quite familiar with. Plants growing in water like Long leaved Barleria (Hygrophila Auriculata), have the innate tendency to eliminate water from their cells. They have been successfully used to cure kidney function deficiency and increase urine output.

We can use the same logic to find out what we might lack and identify the item we need to eat.

Now we shall go deep into the properties of materials found in different atmospheres of the earth.

THRIVING IN WATER

Animals and plants living in water

Fish, shells, crocodile, frog, turtle, oyster, crab, seal, sea weeds, algae and corals are examples. They have evolved in a condition submerged in water and their properties have a built in tolerance and resistance to water and its permeability.

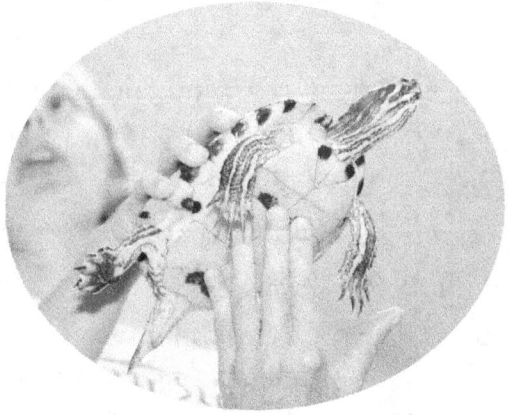

They are capable of extracting nutrients dissolved in water to form concentrates like calcium and mineral deposits. (like shells). They can also accumulate some gummy substances which can repel water.

Many non living substances dissolved in water are also absorbed like salts, minerals or rocks.

Edible materials taken from these sources, for example, fish, algae and salt help the human body to shed excess water and to increase water resistance.

They make our bodies flexible. They make our skins shiny.

Many diseases of the respiratory system are cured by using materials derived from things submerged in water. For example, fish can benefit asthma patients and ashes of corals are used to cure tuberculosis.

Ambergris, an exotic drug collected from the sperm whale is used as an aphrodisiac.

Such materials increase the alkalinity of the body, reduce its acidity, improve vitality and increase its masculinity.

Fresh waters like river and lake

Things found in fresh water are different in many respects to those that are found in the ocean and the seas.

They are softer in texture, gentler in their activities, and their life cycle is comparatively short.

They get enough sunlight even though they are submerged in water.

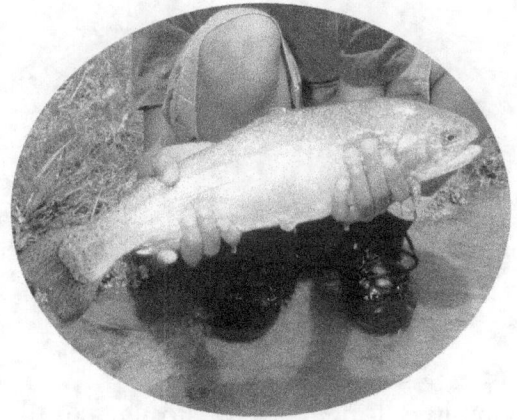

They have more sweet taste and the properties of sweet substances. They too help in reducing excess water in the body.

They act as a tonic while recovering from illness and for building the body.

They are less toxic compared to their counterparts from the sea.

They cool the body and reduce the heat particularly in the stomach.

They act as very good skin and hair conditioners.

They get both abundant water and sunlight.

The foodstuff derived from the rivers and lakes are rejuvenating, body building and soothing to the digestive systems and skin.

Saline water – Sea and Ocean

Sea has saline water which conditions the bodies of animals living in the sea. They are hardened to withstand the corrosion by salts. They are also conditioned to survive in wide temperature variations and turbulent currents.

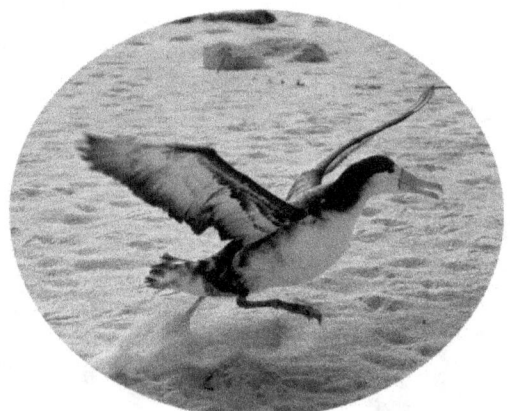

They generally live longer than similar animals living in fresh water.

Most of these life forms live deep under the sea and are exposed to very little sunlight. They get abundant water and electrolytes and some sunlight.

If a person lacks any of these qualities, for example, Vitamin D deficiency, skin problems, accumulation of water in the body for whatever reason, lack of electrolytes, lack of calcium and other minerals, they can find their food from the sea and ocean.

LIVING IN WETLAND

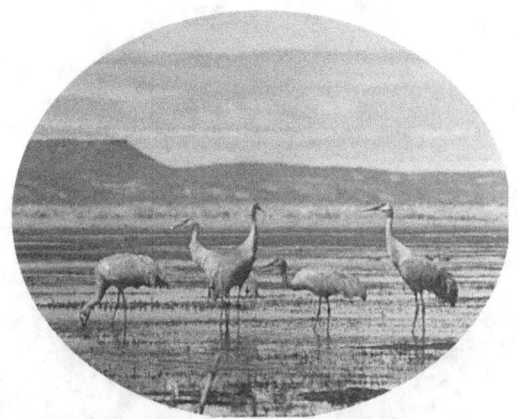

Wetland is a land area that is mostly water logged. It is the soil covered with water and marsh lands can be cited as examples.

Such swamps house a number of organisms and the animals living there have evolved to survive in an atmosphere of moisture and at the same time with access to solid biological substances found on the earth.

In some places the land would be inundated during seasons and the life may be different during such seasons and off-seasons.

They have different profiles.

Their life-cycle is short. Their bodies are conditioned to quickly utilize the nutrition available and grow fast before their life ends in a short span of time when the season changes.

These substances impart a quick response quality to the human body and also offer some immunity boosting properties. They are very useful to persons suffering from general weakness and malnutrition.

DRY-LAND

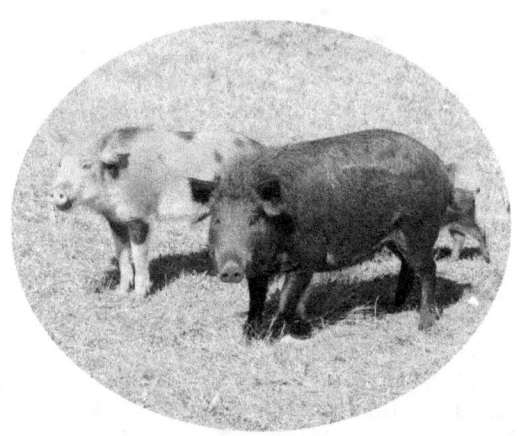

Water is scarce in these areas and rainfall is minimal. The animals and plants know how to conserve water in their bodies. They even save moisture for dry days. They are also fairly resistant to heat and sunshine.

Many life forms are parasites living on other plants and animals.

The foodstuff sourced from these dry land areas help our body to conserve water and bear heat.

They also provide the property to endure hardships and survive in adverse conditions.

They would make good food for convalescing persons elderly persons.

Such foods provide resiliency and flexibility to the human body.

DESERT

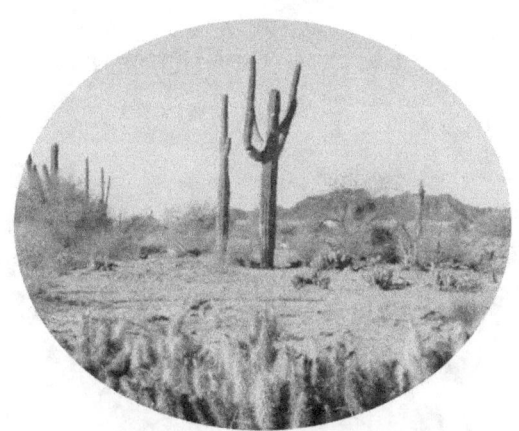

The desert ecosystem is practically dry throughout the year and the life manages to exist in extremely dry and dehydrating conditions.

They not only know how to conserve water but also use less water for their survival. They are hardy.

Very few items found in the desert make good food for humans. A few cactus varieties have been used by tribal societies as medicines.

Aloe Vera is an example of medicinal plant though it is strictly not desert vegetation and grows in semi arid regions as well.

These foods, Aloe Vera in particular, provides the dehydrated human body with the much needed nourishment. People were able to survive long periods of famine and hunger in some countries just by eating Aloe Vera.

It is very good moisturizer for the body and skin. Animals and other plants from desert areas would provide similar benefits.

MOUNTAIN AND FORESTS

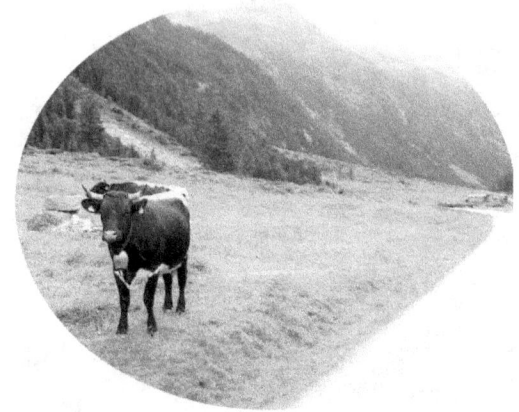

The largest species of plants and animals are found in these areas which are characterised by thick vegetation, frequent rainfalls and adequate sunlight.

There is no dearth of food for the living beings and they have adapted to be choosy about what they eat, and have developed particular patterns in their lifestyle.

They are used to a relatively abundant and protected environment and live a life which is mostly stress free.

They have gone in evolution beyond meeting basic necessities and survival traits.

Food materials derived from these regions contain the properties of finesse and tonality. They would give health overtones to the basic physiological structure.

They are fatty, rich in amino-acids and micro nutrients and provide a rejuvenating property to the body. In a sense, the happiness enjoyed by these animals and plants can be said to be passed on to the humans who consume them.

That is, cells and tissues developed after basic needs are fulfilled form part of the foodstuff from this sector and offer additional benefits to our body.

ICY TERRAINS

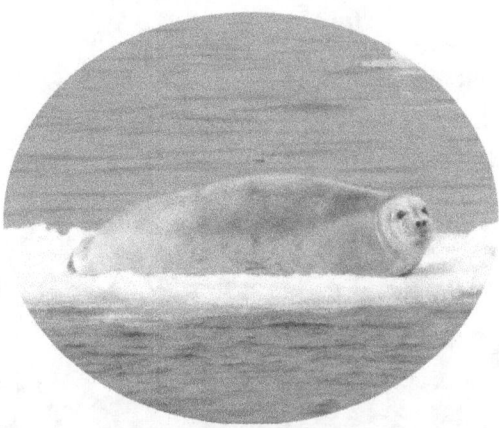

With very little heat available and at freezing temperatures some animals and plants survive in icy areas.

Their bodies have evolved to keep warm and preserve fats which are the opposite of those living in deserts.

Like materials of desert origin, very little foodstuff having special properties can be derived from these areas.

The major ones are fish oils which are good for the skin and the blood circulatory system.

Medicinal plants are not known to exist in such unfavorable circumstances.

Humans use the meat of fish, reindeer and such animals living in icy areas.

Resistance to cold is the major property provided by these food items.

5. SIGNS AND SOLUTIONS

We shall see some conditions frequently encountered by us for which we generally may not go to a physician for advice.

We shall also see how we can solve these problems by some simple techniques.

We will notice that the mind and body are interdependent.

PAIN

Unless the pain or ache is severe and unbearable we may to ignore it. We may take a pill of a popular analgesic and leave it at that. Pain lasts till the stimulus, namely the injury or the disease is healed.

Analgesics and anesthetics help to relieve pain.

Acupuncture is widely used for pain relief.

We can massage the affected part to promote blood circulation and warm it up to relieve the pain.

Counter-irritants like oleo resins of chilly, ginger and pepper have been found to effectively mask pain.

Mental diversion is another tactic used by some.

Eating sweet has shown good results for some especially for children.

TASTE

The tongue can normally sense the taste with accuracy particularly those which are pungent and bitter.

If one feels tasteless of any food, a small dash of a sour fruit juice might help to recover the lost sensation.

Metallic taste can also be cured by citric juices and honey.

Tastelessness may be due to sick health and in that case it gets corrected automatically when the disease is cured.

Lack of taste or alteration of taste due to abuse of tobacco and alcohol or due to intake of very hot food or drink so as to burn the tongue, it will get normal in a few days.

To get a better taste perception it is necessary to crush the food well with teeth and mix completely with saliva while eating them.

This is also a good practice to promote digestion and the accompanying metabolism.

TIREDNESS

If the tiredness is not due to ill health, it can be remedied instantly by taking some sweet stuff and water or juice.

A quick rest or sleep is advisable to reset the body to its normal condition.

Physical tiredness can be relieved by energy drinks and rest while mental tiredness can be cured by relaxation and sleep.

Tiredness of the mind will show symptoms of impatience and irritability along with seemingly tired body.

Diversion of mind is highly successful in regaining strength and enthusiasm.

If enough food was eaten, the body automatically compensates for the lost energy.

IRRITABILITY

Such a temperament can be due to both mental and physical reasons.

Acute diseases of the heart, lungs and vital organs can induce irritability. Sometimes the underlying causes do not show any symptoms at all.

Exclude the possibility of such dangerous illness before tackling irritability.

If it is only a mental problem it can be cured by simple relaxation techniques and eating calming foods.

Foods which are sweet, bland, soft and fresh are calming. Foodstuff that is pungent, spicy, hard and stale are disturbing and not pacifying to irritable persons.

Prudent intake of alcoholic and fruit beverages can be helpful.

Stress relieving lifestyle is absolutely essential to permanently cure irritability.

CONFUSION

It is a condition which results when the thought processes are deadlocked.

It is caused due to inadequate understanding or misunderstanding of the important factors. If the options available are not known one may get confused.

Such kinds of confusion can be sorted out by following mental training exercises.

Confusion sometimes results due to impaired brain function.

Gently massaging the forehead and front part of the head will improve activity of the part of the brain affected by confusion.

A mild stimulant like tea or coffee might help.

Narcotic drugs and alcohol aggravate the problem.

Head should be kept low while sleeping to provide enough blood circulation and rest to the brain and blood vessels of the head and neck.

Deep breathing exercises have also cleared the confused mind in some cases. This is probably due to increased oxygen supply.

Leaving the thinking abruptly and focusing the eyes on a distant object for five minutes has also been helpful, probably by relaxing.

LAZINESS

If it has been the result of physical weakness, nutrition should be enhanced to rehabilitate the person.

Human body gets conditioned by habits and routines. If a person continues to be lethargic for a considerable length of time, then the body adapts itself to such practices and finds itself difficult to cope with sudden hard work.

It is not only a mental problem but also a physiological weakness.

Changing the habits conscientiously can force a schedule on the lazy person and make demands on the body to provide energy at short and enduring times.

In due course, the physiology changes to suit the changed lifestyle.

Foodstuff that is stale, cold and sweet should be avoided and instead hot, spicy and pungent tasting foods should be eaten.

If laziness is solely due to mental reasons it can be solved by proper motivation.

SLEEPINESS

Sleepiness can be due to tiredness, nervous problems, or general weakness.

Accumulation of toxins and wastes in various parts of the body especially in the head is the reason for sleepiness.

Increasing oxygen supply by deep breathing, stimulating blood circulation by mild exercises like walking and energizing drinks may support to overcome sleepiness.

Drastic measures like a cold water bath would harm the body and the brain in particular.

Drinking tea, coffee and hot water infusion of herbs can supplement the waking up.

Cleaning the body of wastes and detoxification are absolutely essential to cure the sleepiness syndrome.

SLEEPLESSNESS

Sleeplessness is primarily caused due to anxiety which may be disguised.

If the mind has an unfinished agenda and a person physically engages in something else, then the mind has not been put off and is still active on the original task.

Such conditions create sleeplessness in a person.

Trying to forcefully sleep or resorting to sleeping pills and other medications would increase the anxiety and would prolong the problem.

Rethinking about the unfinished task and mentally suggesting and believing that the task is finished or suspended without any problem would start the process of relaxation.

Deep breath oxygenation, hot water and aromatic baths, soothing massages, pleasant food and drink, would help.

Alcohol and tobacco would aggravate the problem.

Addition of sweets, nutmeg, and cardamom in the diet also helps.

MEMORY

The human brain is capable of remembering unlimited things. However, when we say we are short of memory, we actually mean that we are not able to retrieve the thing from the storage.

Psychology states that repetition strongly embeds things in to memory and associating one with another helps to recall that from memory.

Our brain uses a pattern recognition system to understands and interpret things.

The best mental training is practice, over and over again.

Physical capacity of the brain is almost the same to all individuals but the way we train our brain is different for each.

One technique may not work for all. Just like habit forming, the brain can be trained by repeating what we prefer to do and avoiding what we do not want to do.

Sweets, food containing salts like Potassium, fresh fruits, vegetables and milk help to improve brain functions.

Sprouted grains, carrots, coriander, and leafy greens and ginger are also beneficial.

Slimy and bland food like, Ladies Finger (Okra), Egg white, gruel or light porridge is good for the brain's health.

CLIMATE TOLERANCE

Resilience to climatic variations can be largely conditioned by the body itself but one's stamina has to endure the transition.

Anybody would be able to adapt to a changed weather condition within a short period of time.

Sudden changes and extreme climates can be harmful to the body. In such cases protective clothing and diet should be maintained till the body gets accustomed to the new atmosphere.

Cold climate requires increased energy to keep warm and fatty foods and carbohydrates will help. Appetizing soups and starters may be necessary to induce hunger and promote digestion.

In hot climates foods gets easily digested and frequent eating may be necessary. The food for hot regions has to be cooling comprising more fruits and vegetables.

Nature has a peculiar way of gifting us with what we need at exactly where we require.

Taking food that is grown or available at our current residence does the trick. That food is surprisingly optimized for the requirements of a person living in that climate and atmosphere.

To get used to a particular climate we need to get used to the food and clothing prevalent in that area.

This would help our body to feel comfortable with that climate.

Another notable point is that we have to consume the food that is normally available during that particular season.

Avoid taking preserved food made of ingredients from another season. It is like wearing winter clothing in summer.

This practice will prevent anyone from getting allergies and illness due to imbalance of the body forces.

EMOTION

Emotions are largely mental expressions but they can be triggered by physiological factors.

For example, alcohol and drugs act not only on the body but also on the mind. Residual effects of drugs, foodstuff, drinks and smoke can be felt for days following their use.

To get normal mental state after an emotional disturbance due to any of the physical factors, one has to reverse the treatment.

This is a complex phenomenon but we can follow a thumb rule to achieve the desired results.

If a food or drug has caused a particular mental reaction, one can take a very small dose (absolutely small so that it won't repeat the previous incident) of the problem stuff over a prolonged period of time (at least ten to fifteen times the time taken originally to consume it) and being conscious of every moment of it.

This action sends a signal to our body about the type of stuff we are putting in and give it adequate time to prepare itself to tackle the coming situation.

This principle is being used in inoculation and vaccination to prevent vulnerability to diseases.

The same holds true in the practice of homeopathy.

So if one was emotional after a particular food, drink or drug, it will help to recreate that condition with only minute controllable quantities of the stuff without taking the risk to repeat the past unpleasant incident.

6. THE INVISIBLE FORCES

The universal elements in the body cannot be seen as they are, but we are able to observe their activities and thus infer their presence.

We so far analyzed the structure and functioning of the physical body and how we can maneuver it to our advantage.

There are invisible forces which also reside in and act in the body which cause the body to function.

Different philosophers and medical practitioners over the time have described these forces in a variety of ways.

They all seem to concur on a basic principle underlying these forces. We shall see them below:

POSITIVE AND NEGATIVE FORCES.

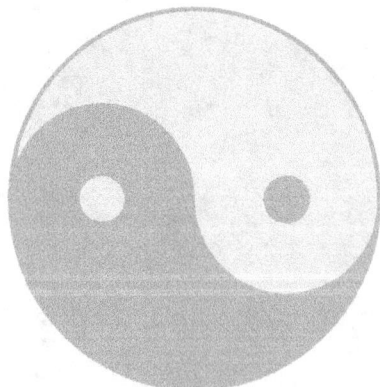

Electricity has both positive and negative forces. The atom has protons and electrons.

Most of the phenomena in the universe are binary - Light and shadow, heat and cold, and so on.

Life forms also comprise of male and female aspects.

Male gender is a human body which contains both masculinity and femininity but wherein the maleness predominates.

The female body has predominantly feminine characteristics. The neutral gender is one which is not decidedly male or female oriented.

The Buddhists call them Yin and Yang.

The Hindus call them as Purusha and Prakruti.

The linguists call them as Vowels and Consonants.

The Chemists call them as Alkali and Acid.

The Alchemists call them as salt and sour.

Whatever you wish to call them it is a fact that the couple exist.

They are like water and soil. The soil is fertile but impotent until water wets it to grow plants.

We shall now see their characteristics.

OPPOSITE AND COMPLEMENTARY.

Male and female aspects are opposite to each other. They are complementary because one is useless without the other. You can observe that nature has a number of examples to demonstrate this equation.

Salt can form only if an alkali and an acid combine. Heat can be understood only relative to cold which is its opposite. There won't be shadow without light.

So we can see that they always go together.

However, their comparative strengths and therefore the individual effects vary.

They both have similar but opposite capabilities. One can neutralize the other.

INTERDEPENDENT FOR EQUILIBRIUM.

Like in magnetism south and north poles attract each other and their magnetic flux attains equilibrium. Like poles repel each other and move until an equal and opposite pole is paired.

Natural attraction of male to female and vice versa demonstrates this.

THE DUALITY OF HUMAN BODY

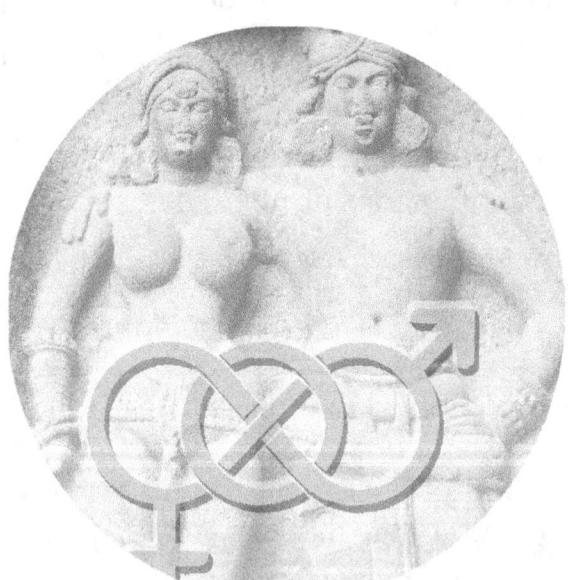

We might observe that men at times behave like women and females too act like males.

We can also see that except for the parts related to reproduction, all the other parts are similar in both male and female bodies.

Let us forget about males and females for the time being and consider the body as a common medium for human beings.

Both the positive and negative charges are present in the body.

The acidic and alkaline radicals are simultaneously active in the body. In our digestive system, for example, saliva in the mouth is alkaline, the enzymes in the stomach are acidic and the ones in intestines are alkaline. This change in pH helps in digesting the food.

Similarly for any of our body's functions both the male and female forces are necessary. The dominance of any one will affect the end result.

COMMON DEFICIENCY AND EXCESS OF THE FORCES

If in a male body feminine forces are dominant or masculine forces are weak, then he will have less manliness and male features.

Facial hair growth, boldness, courage, rational thinking and leadership traits will be lacking.

This condition is caused due to excess acidity in the body. Symptoms may include baldness, digestive disorders, sexual weakness, skin diseases, boils, body heat and desire for sour food or beverage.

Alkaline food, antacids, mineral salts, vegetables, egg white, milk, fat, nuts, bland and slimy food would help to recover from this condition. Sour, hot, spicy food or drinks will aggravate the problem.

Physical exercise would supplement diets in recovery.

Men should be net alkaline to have a powerful body.

Likewise in a female body insufficient feminine forces or excess masculine forces show symptoms like guttural voice, infertility, irregular menstrual periods, facial hair growth, slow actions, lack of emotion and rough mannerisms.

Reducing alkalinity and increasing acidity in the body will reset the balance.

Food and beverage like citrus juices, turmeric, bicarbonate, vinegar and fruits and vegetables in general can be supplemented.

Excess salt and fat should be avoided.

Women should be net acidic to possess a powerful body.

7. Notice to your Body

Who gives the notice? Your five senses.

The senses known as hearing, touch, sight, taste and smell are excellent diagnostic instruments that automatically send their reports for action.

Before any physical discomfort or illness one or more of these instruments notify the body that something is wrong.

They help in preventing many discomforts and diseases. We have to heed to their warnings to maintain a healthy life.

Sight

Good food is nice to look at. One starts to salivate and gets ready to digest such food. The eyes don't generally like bad food. Human beings have been aesthetically decorating food since ages to entice people to eat. We are involuntarily drawn towards attractive food.

The brain remembers the sight when objectionable food was last consumed and warns if such a sight occurs again.

If your eyes don't like a food discard them without fail. If one forcefully eats such food for whatever reason, then the psychology will start to act and complicate the digestive process.

TOUCH

Food that is soft can be cut into small pieces to easily swallow. It can be easily ground in the mouth and in the stomach to extract the nutrients. Hard food is difficult to digest and creates stomach aches and other ailments.

We cook the food to soften them enough to be fit for consumption. Addition of water to the food during cooking is known as hydration. It assists in dissolving the food particles and aids in digestion. Hydrated food is soft and dehydrated food like fries are hard.

The sense of touch can alert us to accept or reject the food. Think twice if the food is hard to cut or chew.

SOUND

Well, sound does not always accompany when we eat food except the crushing sound of our jaws. But it is better to watch out for anything extraordinary like the sound of stone in the dish.

SMELL

The interesting aroma of the food sends signal to the olfactory area of our brain and makes us want to eat it. Good food has good aroma and bad food has bad smell.

It is a very important indicator to decide whether to take or leave a food item. It warns us just before we risk eating something potentially toxic.

Some poisoned food may affect us even if a small bit is tasted. They can indispose a person even if not potent enough to cause a serious health hazard.

It is better to be conservative when we encounter an offensive smell.

TASTE

It will unconditionally determine if the food is good or not. One should never ever disregard its warning.

It will categorically indicate harmful and potentially dangerous foodstuff we may swallow. Food poisoning almost always follows bad taste.

Mouth is the entry point for the food which is intended to build our body tissues.

Taste of materials was dealt at length in the earlier chapter.

Mouth is where we differentiate the tastes and decide about the properties of the foodstuff.

Mouth also recognizes the texture and hardness of the food particle.

We are able to separate undesirable particles from the food in the mouth.

It would be a good practice to always take time to crush and chew the food well in the mouth before swallowing. Unwanted objects like sticks or stones can be eliminated.

The food will be rendered easy for digestion.

The body gets sufficient notice to get prepared for the type of input we are giving.

Prolonged exposure to the taste increases the degree of perceived satisfaction. This is especially good for those who are obese. They can enjoy the food and at the same time reduce the quantity of intake.

8. GOLDEN RULES FOR GOOD HEALTH

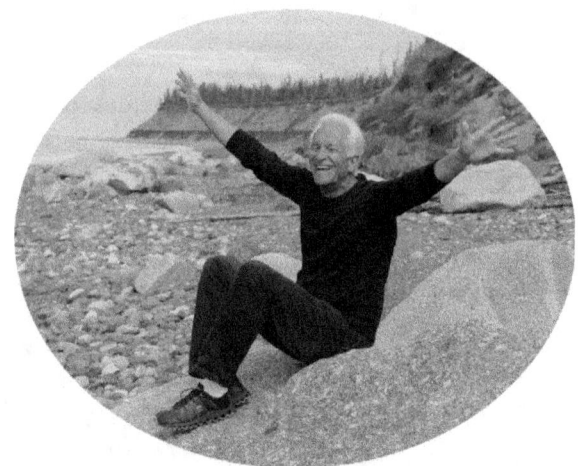

Eating after the previously taken food has been completely digested would avoid the need for any medicines.

We should eat only if we feel hungry. No need to follow a strict regimen.

It will be different from person to person and even for a particular person from time to time.

Digestion is affected by not only physical work but also by mental conditions like stress and ambient weather.

Clean the food in every possible way and then only eat it. Avoid stale food and those not of good quality.

If one eats without limits it is a sure path to ill health.

If I do not know the optimum quantity of food needed for my body I won't also know the amount of disease that I will accumulate.

All input has to be converted in to body tissues or excreted as waste. If anything remains in the body it will breed illness.

It may remain as a solid, liquid or gas and create discomfort.

We should not eat more of a food item if it is extremely good.

Instead we should take time to slowly chew and eat that item to enjoy.

Don't treat the disease alone.

The physician can relieve the symptoms and provide a temporary relief. One has to find out the underlying cause of the disease and correct that problem to get a permanent solution.

The root cause may be our habit, an allergy, the method of preparation, the timing of consumption, imperfect or harmful composition, the ambiance or our psychology.

It may be helpful to find if a pattern is there when the illness occurs.

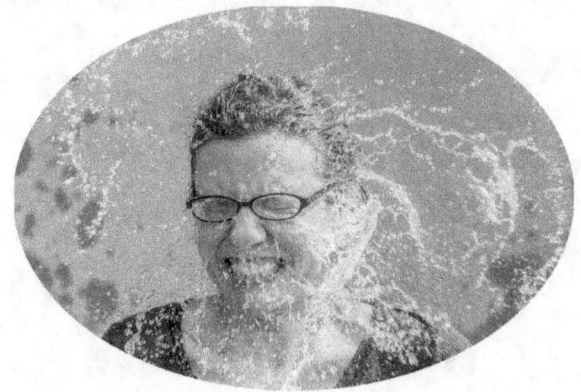

A cool mind creates a cool body.

Learn to relax.

Our mind has an enormous influence on the body. The body blindly accepts what the mind thinks.

A majority of diseases prevalent today like hypertension, heart disease, kidney disease, brain and neurological problems, skin diseases, cough and many others have their origin in stress, perception and other mental reasons.

Learning to maintain calm in adverse situations avoids the above complications.

Learn to concentrate on the task at hand. Distraction increases confusion and breeds stress and dissatisfaction.

Learn to adapt to people and circumstances. It is better to compromise with others than to lose their relationship. Much of stress can be eliminated by good interpersonal relations.

9. MENTAL HEALTH

A healthy mind is more important than a healthy body.

The mind is the driver that drives the vehicle known as the body.

Psychologists have amply demonstrated the beneficial effects we can derive from a positive and proactive mental attitude. Cancer, AIDS and other terminally ill patients have been profoundly benefitted by a confident mind.

Though how the mind controls the body is not clearly known a few facts are worth mentioning.

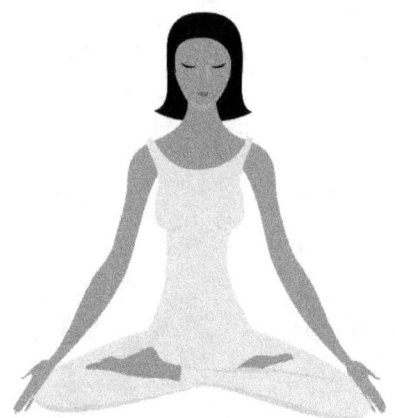

The less work a mind does, the less stressed the mind is, the slower it functions effectively concentrating on the core task.

This is termed as meditation. In these circumstances there is less demand for energy.

The heart and lungs do less work as evidenced by reduced breathing and heart rates during meditation.

Less work for the vital organs prolongs lifespan.

Is it true?

Animals like tiger, horse and dogs grow fast, run fast, breathe fast and die fast.

A flying ant species grows so fast its life is just a day.

One of the slowest animals, the tortoise lives for about three centuries. It breathes very slow compared to most of the animals.

Slow breathing correlates well with longevity.

Meditation is a training of the mind to relax, concentrate and increase awareness.

While meditation is very effective in the long term to enhance mental potential some short term solutions are also required in our daily lives.

Consistent stable breathing calms the mind. A deep breath pacifies tension.

Increased oxygen relieves tiredness of the brain.

Whatever may be the reason, we are not interested in theory but it is a fact that shallow breathing has been found to calm the mind.

So when in disturbed state of mind one should do some breathing exercise or at the least go out to a natural surrounding and inhale fresh air.

Straining the body while the mind is stressed effectively counters mental tension.

Doing some physically demanding work actually relieves stress.

Engaging in sports, gardening, playing with kids and walking pets are very effective seasoning the mind.

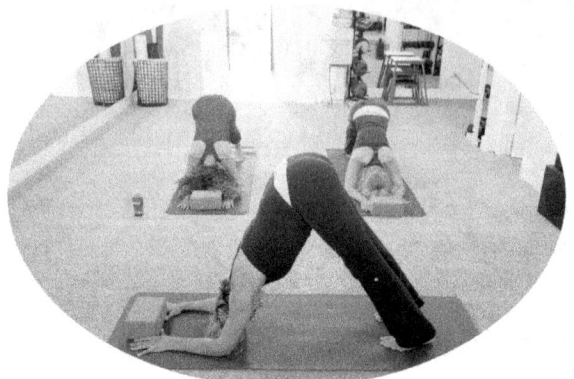

The mindset is the foundation on which all our thinking is based.

One should be positive and confident.

We should avoid all negative thoughts that divert our potential energy away from productive uses and spends them in useless activities.

The right attitude stems from the right mindset.

POWER YOUR BODY

10. SUMMARY

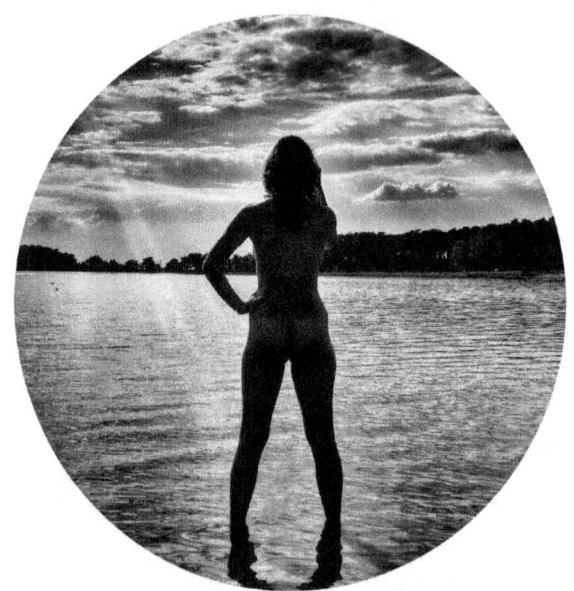

We took a different approach to analyze the body and categorize it into three agile divisions.

We also studied about how they interact among themselves and maintain equilibrium. The effects of imbalance of these elements and the common scenarios encountered by us were also seen.

We interpreted the structure of the life that is present in the body to understand how it functions and to keep ourselves in harmony with it.

We studied how food is an important factor for good health and how it affects our body and mind.

We also saw how we can manipulate foodstuff selection to achieve our desired results.

We found that the sense of taste can be a very useful tool to identify the characteristics of different foodstuff.

Thus by internally observing our body we can diagnose and cure most of our illness and improve the wellbeing.

We also saw what were the characteristics of substances originating from different atmospheres are and how they affect our health.

We studied about simple solutions to common mental and physical problems based on the signs shown by them.

We analyzed the invisible forces in the body that are common to all life forms and how they function in the human body.

Notification mechanisms of the senses and how they forewarn us of impending diseases were also seen.

We saw the workings of the mind and how it has an influence on the body and it's potential.

To power your body without sacrificing your lifestyle you simply follow your own body's messages.

Do what you are comfortable with, eat what you like but that is also good for you, avoid what you don't like and that is bad for you, exercise as you can or prefer and lead a happy life.

The only rule is pay attention to your body's messages.

Your mind, your body and you are unique and only you can master them.

ABOUT THE AUTHOR

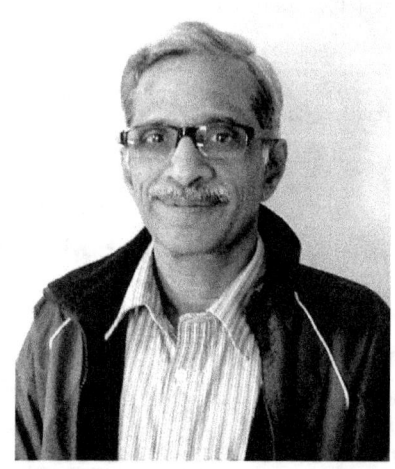

The author has three decades of real life experience in health, diet, wellness, herbs, alternative therapies, yoga, meditation, culture, spirituality and personal consultation.

The author is passionately curious to understand everything in this universe and hence his pen name Curion.

His writings reflect his thinking, experiences and explorations about powering your body in the most comfortable and natural way. It means being yourself. Relaxed and feeling safe!

His study and experience shows you how to easily maintain good health. Your perception of your body will be quite different when you finish reading his works.